Commit with Confidence

The Lactation Reference Guide

Author:

PierreMarie Vital

Certified Breastfeeding Specialist

ISBN: 978-0578948126

2nd Edition

TABLE OF CONTENTS

Images captured by Ellie Stover,
primary photographer for
MidHudson Chocolate Milk.

COMMIT WITH CONFIDENCE WAS WRITTEN AS A SUPPORT TOOL NOT A REPLACEMENT FOR PERSONALIZED CARE.

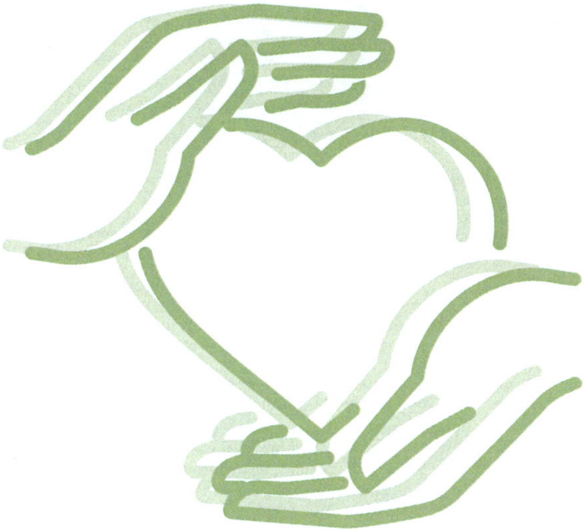

At any point, if you feel overwhelmed or distressed on your journey,
PLEASE seek support.
you deserve it!

Lactation is a language of Love

How do you feel about your upcoming journey?

Educating yourself is a huge step.

Be proud of wanting to learn how to best support your growing family.

/MATERNAL MENTAL HEALTH/

Is the recognition that sustaining and supporting life broadens an individual's emotional landscape.

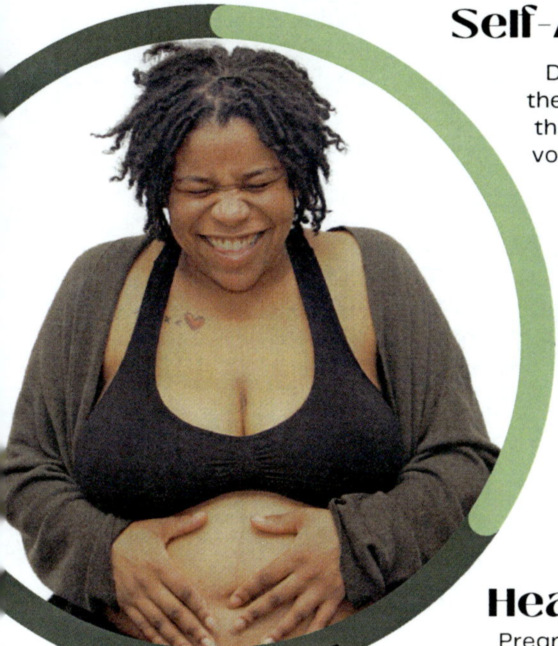

Captured by: Jordan Coburn

Self-Advocacy

During pregnancy a person is introduced to the responsibilities of parenting through how they manage their journey. When we use our voice we are placing our influence towards a particular ideas and acknowledging the validity of those ideals.

Honor Journey

We refer to pregnancy as a journey because the outcome even at its best is unknown. Honoring the pregnancy journey means to exalt and examine all the emotions that present themselves during the transformative process. .

Heals Wounds

Pregnancy alters the body by realigning bodily systems to provide maximum nutrients and optimum safety for the growing child. This process also exposes emotional attachments and can be a well of personal growth and grounding strength.

Empowerment

Supporting your child throughout pregnancy and guiding them safely through their birth is incredibly empowering. The objective of emotional support is for the parent to trust in their power and ability as a navigator.

HUMAN MILK BENEFITS

The placenta is an organ that your body grows to sustain your child while you're pregnant. After your child enters the world, your placenta will detach and will arrive shortly after delivery. The placenta detaching Lactogenesis II, which is the formal name for milk production.

As you initially begin your postpartum journey your body receives signals to secrete milk it began formulating during your 2nd trimester. Hormones like oxytocin aid in postpartum recovery. Oxytocin causes uterine contractions and helps shrink the uterus back to its pre-pregnancy size.

Your colostrum is the initial sticky yellow liquid you'll be expressing. Your milk is the most nutrient-dense food for your child, since it contains a wide variety of proteins, vitamins, in addition to fats and immunity boosting properties.

Providing milk and engaging in skin-to-skin contact strengthens brain stimuli by creating healthy emotional connections. As your child transitions outside of the womb they'll explore in curiosity feeling safe in their new environment.

HUMAN MILK BENEFITS

When a routine is established, producing milk is an easy and efficient method of feeding your child. Human milk does not have the same financial burden as artificial milk. It does cost because your time is valuable and you engage in physical and emotional labor.

Your child's latch will communicate their needs and your body will adjust the composition of your milk. It's important to understand that latching helps develop certain bodily functions like jaw mobility and dexterity.

Producing milk long-term has tremendous health benefits for both parent and child. Including lowering the risk of developing certain cancers, hypertension, and diabetes.

Human milk is easier to digest than formula, which means less discomfort when passing gas and better-smelling diapers.

Lactation as a discipline is the most sustainable feeding choice. It reduces many of the stressors placed on the environment and is an investment in communal wellness.

HUMAN MILK COMPOSITION

Human milk is 87% WATER. It is important to remember with newborns that water by itself does not have the nutrient value babies need, and with such small stomachs introducing water too young can cause discomfort.

Human milk contains a mix of vitamins and minerals that help build strong bones, make red blood cells and help muscles and nerves function properly.

Human milk contains lactose which is a complex carbohydrate that provides the energy necessary for brain development. It is also rich in Omega 3s and complex lipids, whey, casein and nucleotides to promote growth and development. The HAMLET protein-lipid complex is also present in human milk which helps protect against approximately 40 types of cancer. Human milk also contains stem cells which help repair the body.

Human milk contains immunoglobulins, which are antibodies that fight bacteria, viruses, fungus and parasites.

Human milk has hormones that assist with growth and development. Some help regulate blood pressure and metabolism and while some help relieve pain and reduce stress.

PROLACTIN

Prolactin is released when the nipple is stimulated by the suckling motion. The hormone Prolactin creates feelings of calmness and a yearning to connect with your child. Infrequent feedings can lower prolactin levels and decrease supply. Prolactin levels are higher between the hours of 12am-5am, expressing milk between those hours can help establish a healthy supply.

OXYTOCIN

Oxytocin causes the muscles around the alveoli to contract and initiate the process commonly known as the "let-down". Oxytocin levels rise when a new parent sees, smells, looks, or even thinks about their baby. The hormone Oxytocin also promotes uterine contractions, helping control postpartum bleeding and decreasing the puffiness of the uterus.

MILK TRANSITIONS

Colostrum

Colostrum is the first stage of your milk supply. The thick sticky yellow liquid is high in body-building proteins and nutrient-packed minerals. Your body will produce colostrum in small amounts because your baby's stomach is still very small.

Transitional

Between days 3-8 your milk will become rich in water soluble vitamins. Your milk will now begin to increase in lactose in fat as your baby begins to regain general weight loss (up to 10% of their birth weight) and actively begin to acclimate to their environment.

Mature

Approximately 10 - 14 days after birth your body will be producing mature milk. Mature milk reflects the nutrient intake of the producing parent and the stimulus of the nursling. To build a steady supply of milk it is important to nurse on demand (approximately 8-12x a day) or pump every 2-3 hours, it can take up to six weeks for your supply to regulate.

LACTATION MYTHS

If I have smaller breasts, I won't produce enough milk

No matter your cup size, you should be confident in your ability to supply enough milk for your child.

I'll have to maintain a strict diet

You can eat whatever you want! To help maintain your energy eat nutrient dense foods stay hydrated.

It's supposed to hurt.

Pain is a sign that something should be addressed and corrected.

Nursing will make me saggy.

Skin stretches during pregnancy and with time. Learning to embrace the power of your body beyond its appearance is one of the ways lactation helps us develop body autonomy.

WHAT IF

I'm a survivor of sexual assault and/or abuse?

Lactation is a great way to develop a form of sovereignty or power over our experiences. It is important to discuss with your support system your feelings towards pending physical interactions with your child. Seek professional help to assist you in sorting through the complexity of your feelings.

My family and friends do not support me?

If you desire, you can take the time to educate your support system on the benefits of lactation. Invite them to the spaces you've found so they can understand more about why you are so passionate about producing milk. It is important to remember this is your choice and journey.

My partner seems uncomfortable?

Take the time to help your partner understand the commitment you are making to your growing family. Let them know that they are vital to your postpartum success and that there are several ways for them to still be involved. If they complain that your physical relationship will suffer, it is important to remind them that this time is for your body to heal. and for you to process the power you've embraced.

CAN I

PRODUCE MILK if I've had A c-section

Of course! Your body has been making milk throughout your pregnancy. Individuals who have had a belly birth can produce milk by taking proactive measures. such as observing the golden hour as long as there is no medical emergency.

PRODUCE MILK for multiples

Many parents of multiples produce milk for their children. Tandem nursing is a goal and it's okay if it takes time, your children will develop skills at their own rate. Feeding babies one after another helps them develop a routine and helps you establish a supply that will ultimately be their primary source of nutrition.

PRODUCE MILK if my child is premature

Depending on how early your warrior is born will determine whether you can attempt latching. However, your body will receive the signal that gestation has been completed and it is now time to provide sustenance for your little one on the outside. Follow a newborn feeding schedule and pump every 2-3 hours and ask the hospital for a pump so you can begin producing milk as soon as possible. Don't forget to inquire about donor milk!

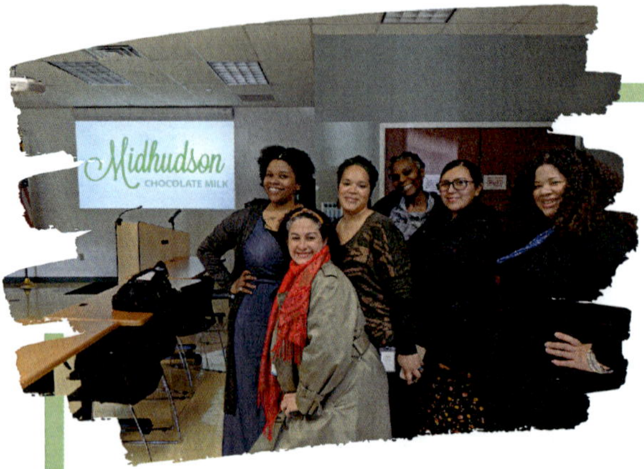

WHERE DO I TURN TO FOR SUPPORT ?

Professionals

IBCLC's, CBS's and CLC's are credentialed professionals who specialize in lactation. These private practice healthcare professionals create customized care plans to support you in your lactation journey. Doulas's will also often invest in lactation support training

Community resources

WIC has individuals on staff that has personally engaged in lactation and are trained to assist called Breastfeeding Peer Counselors. They provide general support and assistance for active WIC participants.

Support spaces

Groups like R.O.S.E. Breast Friend program, Chocolate Milk Cafe, BabyCafe, Postpartum Support International, and La Leche League offer wonderful support groups that offer you the opportunity to connect and learn alongside other parents. The iRTH, Meet Akina, and Peanut app are also great perinatal and support resources. These spaces are often filled with professionals and peers

LET YOUR SUPPORT SYSTEM

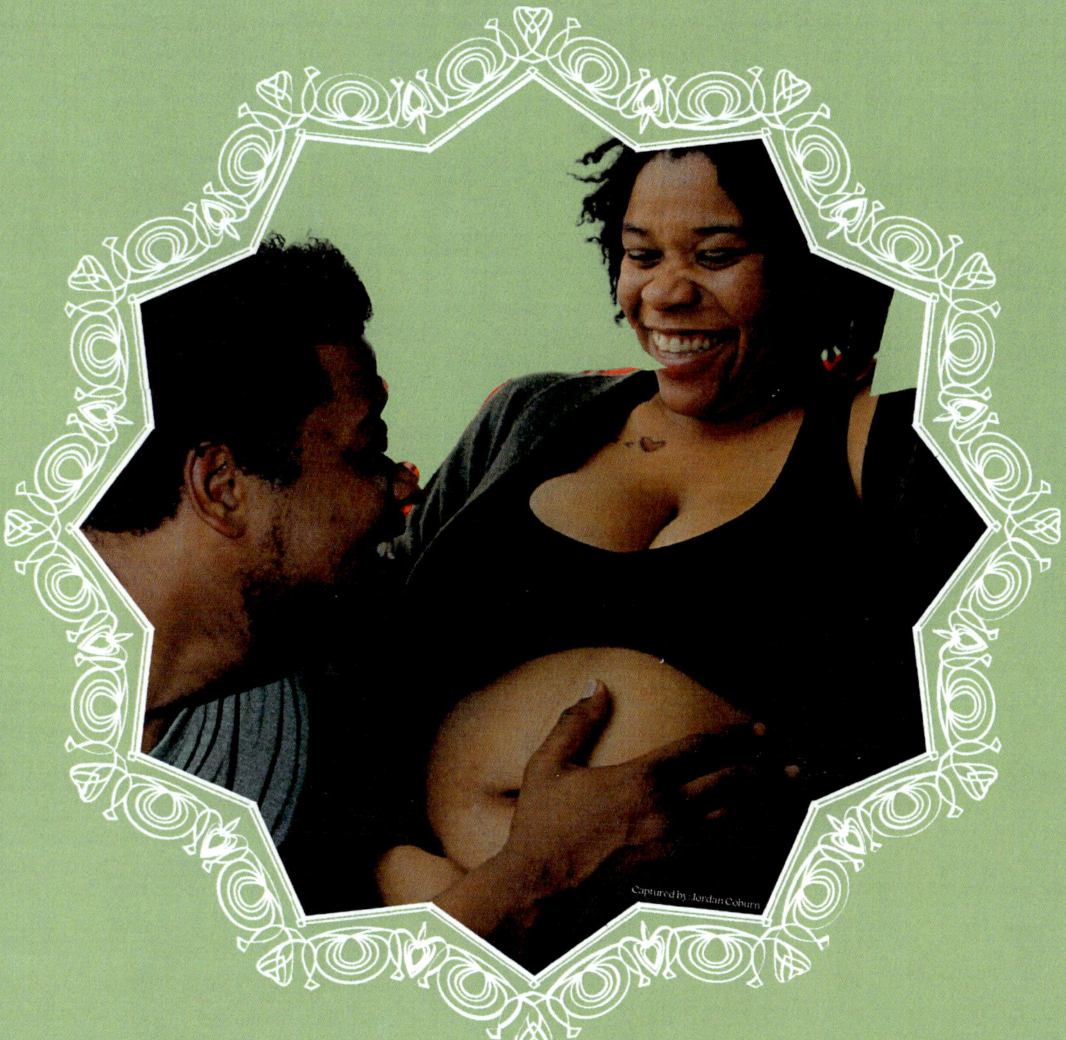
Captured by: Jordan Coburn

SUPPORT YOU!

PREPARING FOR YOUR HOSPITAL BIRTH

Have a birth plan and make sure that it states your desire to give your baby the milk you produce first. Make sure it states no formula be introduced without your expressed consent, and that pacifiers are not used to avoid nipple confusion as you begin your journey.

Most hospitals and birthing centers encourage you to register in advance, if that isn't possible have your insurance card packed in your hospital bag.

Being prepared to relieve discomfort are great ways to encourage a low-stress birth. Counter pressure and aromatherapy are effective ways to provide pain relief.

Be prepared! You may be confined to the birthing center or even your delivery area, having your charger will keep you connected to family and snacks will help avoid stress from lack of sustenance.

Lip balm is great for dry lips from all the breathwork during labor. Honey sticks are a compact source of high energy and don't forget your toiletries.

Pack loose clothing, your birth experience, and your initial days postpartum will be all about low impact and slow movements.

Golden Hour Observance

The Golden Hour is the term used when the newly postpartum parent and their child engage in skin-to-skin contact undisturbed for approximately 60-90 minutes.

Observing the golden hour encourages healthy postpartum recovery by letting the body naturally begin the process of healing. The practice also improves your child's ability to regulate to their new environment.

The vernix caseosa is a off-white waxy coating that protects babies in the womb from infectious diseases. Engaging in skin to skin immediately after birth allows for the vernix to permeate the skin as an additional layer of protection.

The breast crawl is when your newborn recognizes the scent of amniotic fluid being secreted from glands on the area surrounding your nipple. Your darkened nipples provide a deep contrast that your newborn can identify despite their hazy black and white vision.

LET'S TALK LATCH

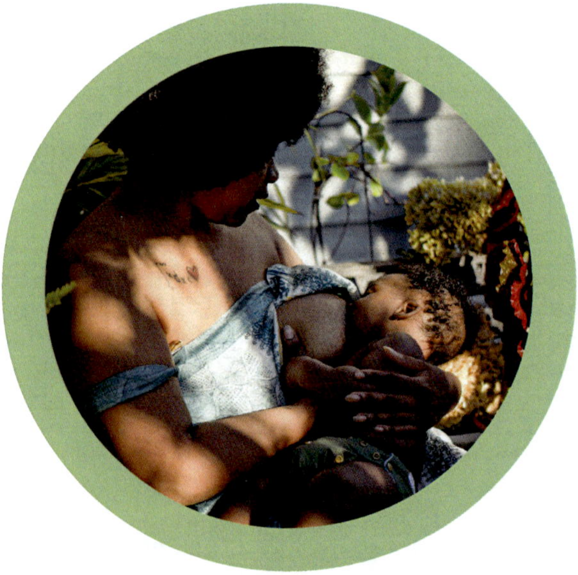

Securing a deep latch is essential if you want to nurse.

A shallow latch can cause extreme discomfort and disrupt your milk supply by pinching nerve endings in the nipple.

Remember it is breast/chest feeding not nipple feeding.

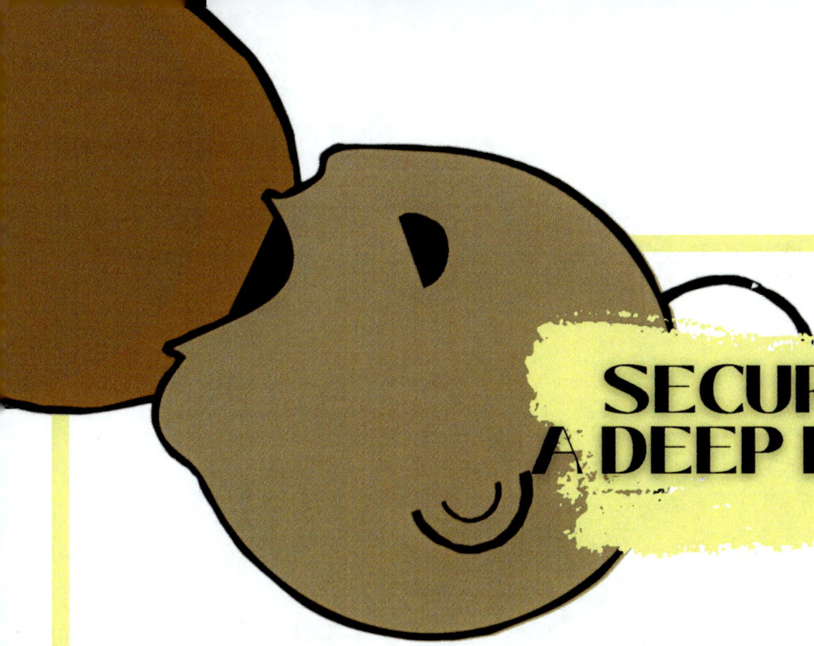

SECURING A DEEP LATCH

Expressing some milk before attempting to latch baby can help your nipple remain erect for latching and stimulate your letdown reducing the initial amount of work for your child to do.
See Hand expression on page 28.

It is important you are in a relaxed position. Do not try to stretch your breast, bring baby to your nipple. Gravity is your friend! Do not try to have your milk compete against a natural flow.

When positioning your baby make sure they are facing you, that their head is turned towards your chest and that their stomach is facing your stomach.

Align your child's nose in the direction of your nipple. Naturally, their head will try to recline fully back. Allow them to lean gently as you support their neck. Their jaw should relax allowing you to guide the areola into their mouth. Point your nipple towards your child's nose so that the bottom half of your areola is also a part of their area to latch.

When successfully latched their lips should be flared outward creating suction around the areola not clenched around the nipple. Once they begin to remove milk their ears and jaw will move rhythmically, you'll be able to hear the 'suck, pause, swallow' pattern of a deep latch.

DO NOT forcibly pull your nipple out of your child's mouth while they're actively latched. It can cause sharp pain and/or result in nerve damage. If you'd like to end a session gently insert your index finger into your child's mouth and slowly rock it back and forth breaking the tension of their latch. After a nursing session your nipple should be round. If your nipple is slanted or has a white line across the latch is not deep enough and it may cause pain.

NURSING HOLDS

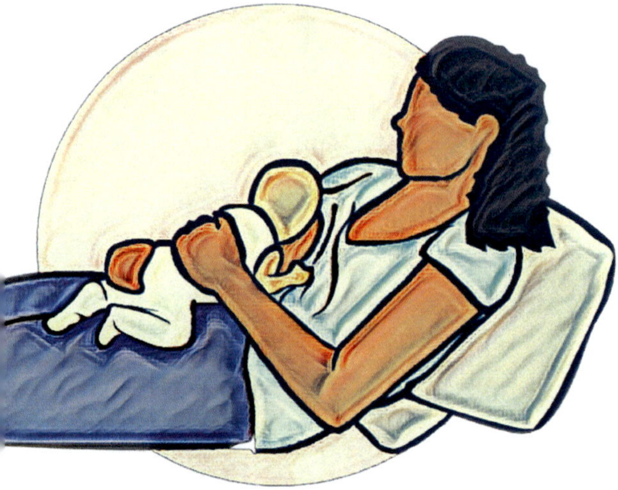

Laid Back

Laid back is a slightly reclined position with head and shoulders supported by a comfortable pillow. Lay your baby on you, stomach to stomach with their head positioned next to your breast. From here you can assist them with latching comfortably.

Side-Lying

Both you and baby lie down on your side facing each other. Make sure their stomach is also facing inward. Make sure the bed is clear of any hazards before you lay down and be aware that you may fall asleep in this position.

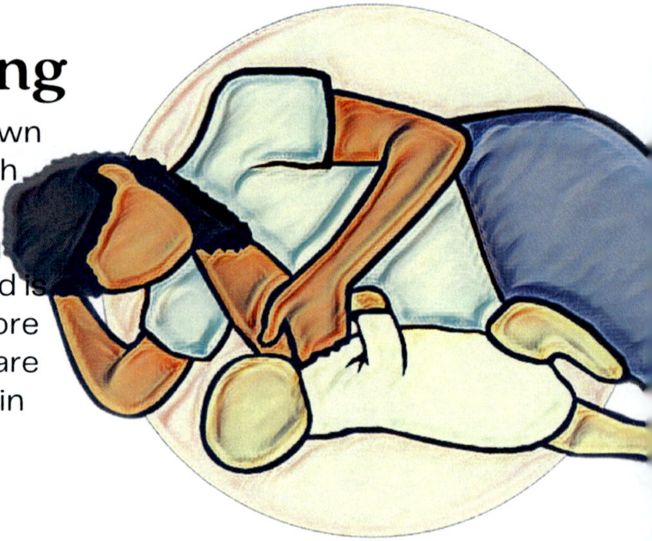

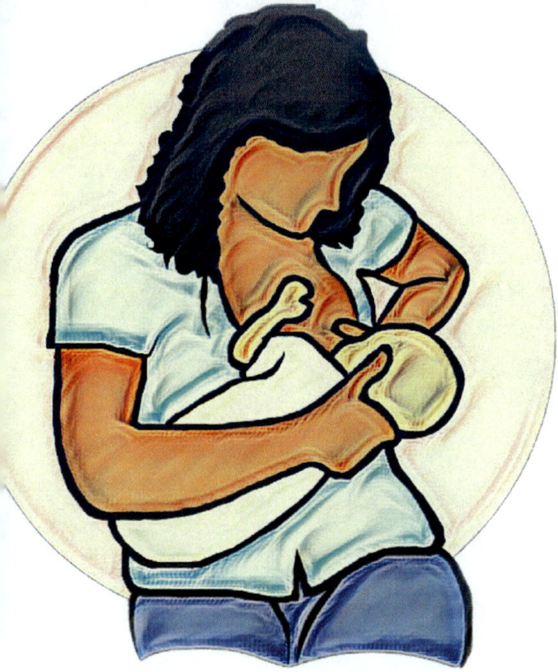

Cross Body

The crossbody hold is similar to the cradle hold. However, the opposite arm of the side in use is where the baby is supported. This frees the hand on the opposite side to massage the breast; aiding milk production.

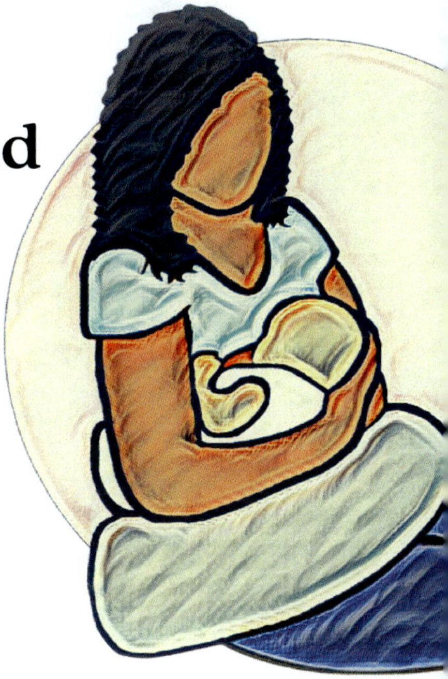

Football Hold

Baby is positioned against the side of your body, with their body wrapping around your side, stomach facing inward. The hand on the side of the breast in use supports the baby by the neck. The other hand is used to assist the baby with latching, and if necessary massage to help stimulate a let-down.

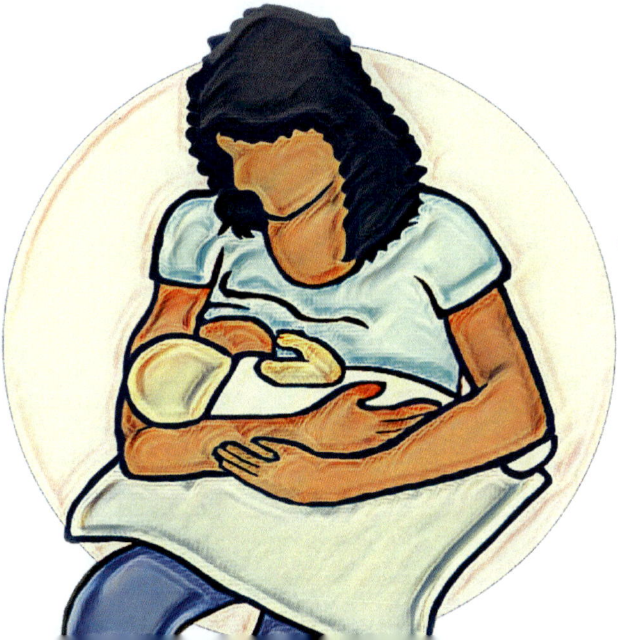

Cradle Hold

In the cradle hold, the baby is lying on their side across your lap supported by a pillow, their head cradled by the arm they are nursing from.

MILK EXPRESSION IS LACTATION!

Reasons a person may pump...

- **Premature Birth**
- **Severe Feeding Issues**
- **Separated from Infant**
- **Attending School**
- **Returning to Work**

Or sometimes it is simply better for the relationship of the parent and baby, whatever the reason, pumping is an enriching lactation journey.

If you are exclusively nursing for the first few weeks it is important to wait until your supply is established before you begin pumping. Pumping too soon can create an oversupply and can result in engorgement.

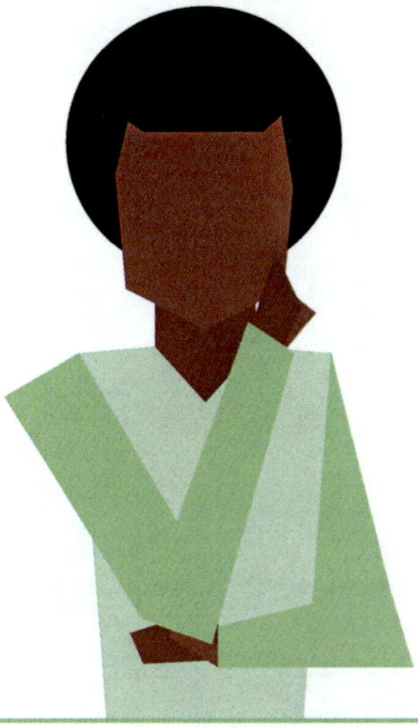

WHAT TO CONSIDER WHEN CHOOSING A PUMP?

Cost.
Does my insurance offer options?

Durability.
How often will I be pumping?

Style.
What will be my pumping environment?

Suction.
How efficient is the unit?

Clean.
What maintenance does the unit require?

Most insurance companies provide new parents milk removal systems. Contact your insurance provider during your 3rd trimester to find out what options they have available and if they cover any replacement parts.

LEARNING YOUR PUMP

Learning how to use your pump properly and effectively is important to efficient milk removal, which ensures a steady supply. Review the instructions and familiarize yourself with the pump and its settings. Check if your flange is the appropriate size. It should not constrict your nipple or have gaps on either side. It's important to wash your hands and ensure your pump parts such as flanges and bottles are clean before use.

Before you begin, make sure you are in a comfortable position. Having a picture or video of your child will promote oxytocin flow as well as a blanket they were recently wrapped in. A gentle massage or applying some warmth can also help encourage your milk to flow. Stimulating your nipples to imitate the rooting sensation also can promote prolactin production.

LEARNING YOUR PUMP

Insurance companies sometimes offer additional pump parts and accessories for free! For more convenient pumping ask your insurance company if they offer a hands-free pumping device, for free or at a discount. There are also pumping bras to convert an electric unit into a hands-free unit. DiY tutorials for adapting other items like sports bras, postpartum underwear, and tank tops are available on YouTube and Pinterest.

Before attaching the flange you can lightly lubricate the funnel portion to create a tighter seal. Start with a slow suction to replicate the feeding pattern of a newborn. Slowly increase speed for a higher rate of suction, but never to the point of discomfort. Pump for up to 20 minutes on each side or until the milk stops flowing. Take your time when you detach your flanges and bag your milk for storage. Some individuals store pump parts attached to the storage bottle as they collect throughout the day, and store their milk at once.

Common Milk Expression Issues

Clogged Ducts

Much like engorgement clogged ducts occur when milk isn't removed consistently. Milk will gather in the ducts and cause a disruption with the flow or a blockage. The clogged duct(s) will be slightly raised areas where you can feel the milk pooling. Unlike engorgement clogged ducts are in specific areas and require direct care. When removing clogged milk, direct their latch and align their nose with the direction of the clogged duct, this allows for a deep latch directly on the impacted duct. Dangle feeding with a directed latch also allows gravity to help your child remove the clogged milk. Gentle hand expression can also be done as well as using the included milk catcher. Additionally, you can add half a TBSP of Epsom salt to approximately ½ warm water and follow included directions to properly secure the silicone hand pump. The suction of the milk catcher in addition to Epsom salt can help draw out the clogged milk. You can use gentle massaging or use a vibrating device on the affected area to help loosen the trapped milk.

If not treated, clogged ducts can develop into an infection called mastitis which requires antibiotics. In extreme cases, the infection will set in and create an abscess that requires surgery for removal.

It's important to make sure you empty your breasts readily to maintain your supply and stay healthy.

Common Milk Expression Issues

Leaking

As your supply regulates you may find yourself leaking at random times. This is normal and will not last for the duration of your lactation journey. Crossing your arms and pressing gently can create counter pressure to help stifle the flow. Placing a towel underneath you while you sleep can help avoid discomfort along with washable or disposable nursing pads.

Sore Nipples

As we've discussed you are not supposed to experience pain. Soreness is just a mild tenderness due to the amount of usage your nipples are receiving. The soreness will not continue for the remainder of your journey.

Engorgement

The increase of milk can lead to an uncomfortable pressure called engorgement. To relieve engorgement it's best to express some milk, you can take a warm shower, hand express, or use a silicone milk catcher or a Thera-gel compress to apply warmth. It's important to continue intentional milk removal to relieve the inflammation of engorgement. Getting on all fours with a baby positioned to latch is called dangle feeding. This process allows gravity to assist in milk removal. If you feel the swelling or inflammation of engorgement is deterring you from continuing apply a cool compress in intervals until the discomfort subsides. As your supply regulates the likelihood of this lessens unless you go long periods without expressing milk.

HAND EXPRESSION

- Wash your hands to maintain a safe environment for your child. Take the time to acknowledge any doubts you have and wash them away.

- Make sure you are in a comfortable environment. a seated relaxed position allows gravity to assist in the flow of your milk.

- Before attempting to hand express, a gentle lymphatic massage can increase milk flow. Place one hand atop a breast, fingers facing your armpit and the other hand cradling the breast from underneath. Gently apply pressure massaging in a circular pattern, making your way to the sides, repeat as comfort allows.

- To begin expressing, make a C-shape with your thumb on top using your right hand if expressing the left breast. You can use the same hand making the C-Shape or your free hand to gently massage your breast with low impact and slow movements.

- maintain the c-shape when going to engage in milk expression and lightly pull your fingers towards your chest. take this time to look for areas you'd like to concentrate on for expression.

- gently apply pressure as you move your fingers down towards the nipple. as you express milk your fingers should not lift from the breast ending at the base of the nipple.

- DO NOT pinch your nipple trying to squeeze milk and DO NOT rub the skin on your breasts trying to force milk expression.

- Short frequent sessions similar to the newborn feeding schedule will stimulate the body to produce more milk. In the beginning, the process is generally 20-30 minutes from set up to clean up.

HUNGER CUES

In the womb your child did not need to ask for any anything, so with limited verbal communication they'll be able to give you cues when they are hungry.

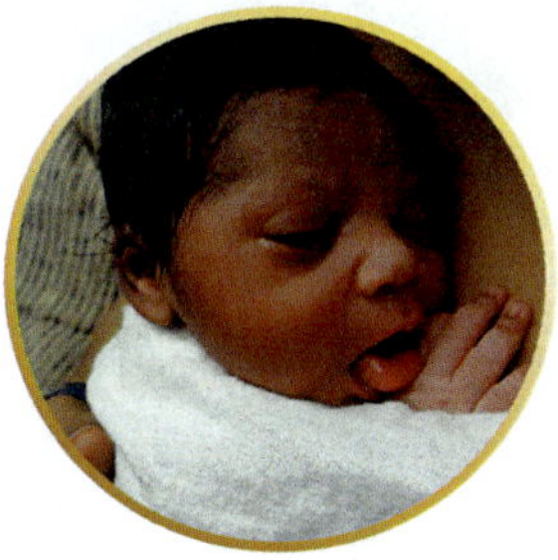

Newborn babies respond to the expansion of their environment by exhibiting a startle reflex that is often triggered by new sensory experiences. However, when your child begins stirring, the motion is them adjusting to the call of hunger. After their initial stirring, they'll begin to bring their hands to their mouth or stick their tongue out. They may also bob their head, "rooting" or searching for food since they've expressed their desire to be fed. Once a baby is crying they are annoyed. Crying is a sign of distress and is the last cue your child will present.

Your baby may eat often, adjusting to their new environment requires a lot of energy. It may be tiring adjusting to your newborn's schedule. Staying nourished, hydrated, and maintaining a low-stress level will help with the transition. Ask for help when it's possible, you deserve the support!

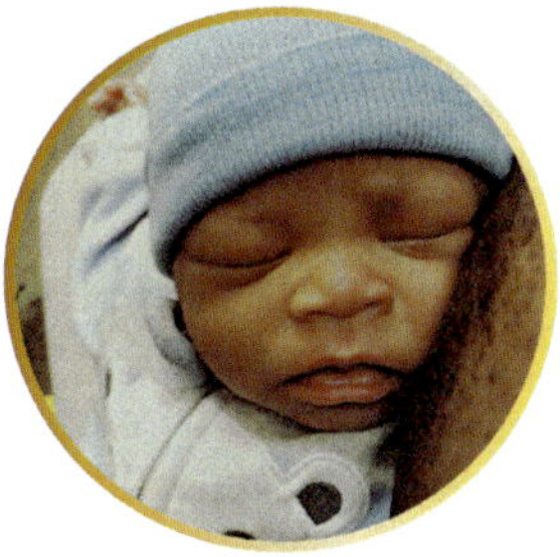

Baby will show obvious signs of relief and contentment when they are full. Their fingers, hands, legs will become relaxed. They may relax their arms over their chest. They will passively suckle or may let go of the breasts completely

PARTNER SUPPORT

During the postpartum period the body transitions into a new phase of engagement. Organs are shifting back; wounds are healing, and hormones are in flux. Simple acts like massaging joints, running a foot bath, and feeding the new parent are impactful interactions that provide relief.

In the womb, babies do not have to release gas, So outside of the womb, many babies are uncomfortable learning to do so. Burping a baby or pumping their legs to release gas is a great way for your partner to engage the baby and foster trusting relationships.

Water can help calm babies by reminding them of the womb, A bath is a great way for your partner to share in the responsibilities of parenting. Storytime, soothing scents, and comforting motions is a great way to build a relationship with your new baby.

PARTNER SUPPORT CONTINUED

The transition outside of the womb is jarring in many ways for your newborn. Having them lay on your partner's chest, skin to skin is a great way to help them thrive. The constant embrace helps regulate the baby's temperature, stabilizes bodily functions, and aids in brain development. Melody and rhythm help maintain your child's attention while introducing them to the complexity of sound outside of the womb. The actual vibrations from your voice help regulate their heartbeat and also stimulate brain development.

Let your partner know you value their encouragement and that it helps you travel confidently in this experience. Learn about the basics together, review this guide with your partner so they can learn helpful tips, such as various holds and how to secure a deep latch. When you and your support system are informed you can be more proactive than reactive to any obstacles.

VILLAGE SUPPORT POSTPARTUM

Inform any visitors to respect whatever environment you'll need to practice latching and nursing your child. They'll nurse often, so learning their cues and understanding developmental expectations will help you gain confidence on your journey.

Exhaustion happens easily with a newborn baby, let your family know that you don't have the energy to "entertain company" for long. Hopefully they'll understand that you just performed magic and require time to recharge as you love on your newborn

Calling ahead goes a long way with how receptive we are with others during their visit. Remind family that calling ahead will give you time to prepare. Whether it is so you can change clothes or simply take a couple of deep breathes, the chance to prepare eases the pressure of "entertaining" company.

No lingering odors or lotions. A newborn baby is incredibly sensitive to their new environment. Scents and lotions carry ingredients that may be overwhelming for baby. Remind family that it is best to visit them au naturale.

The first 6 weeks postpartum include several adjustments and transitions for everyone in the home. Preparing and cooking meals is hard with the demanding schedule of a newborn. Let your family know you'd appreciate meals or gift cards so there is one less stressor while growing into your new role.

When people visit they may offer to help you, take the help you deserve. It's okay to remind company they are there to help YOU not baby. Ask for assistance with chores that may be neglected or to prep your space for ease throughout the day.

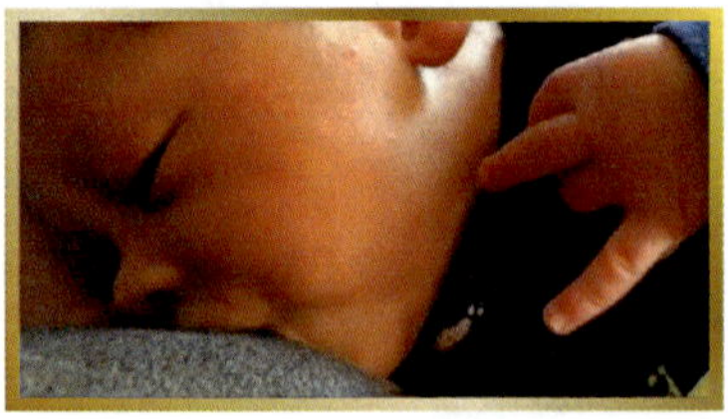

THE FIRST FEW WEEKS

Protein rich foods such as sweet potatoes and spinach help the body repair wounds and rejuvenate during postpartum recovery. A nutrient rich diet is essential to maximize the benefits of your milk.

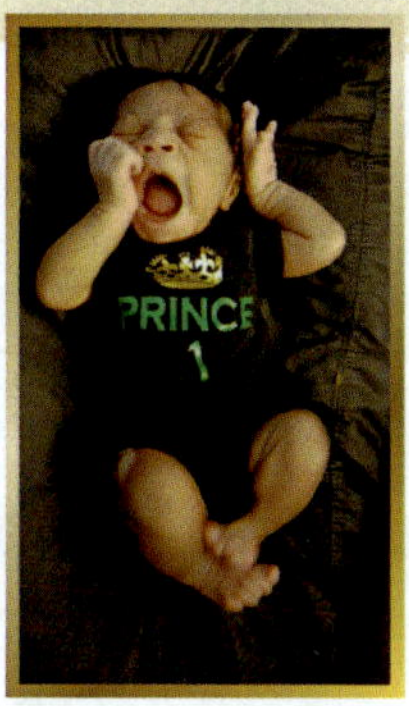

Your newborn will grow quickly, but it's important to keep in mind how small their stomachs are to keep a realistic expectation of their milk consumption.

Tracking soiled diapers is a great way to gauge whether your child is getting enough to eat. Ideally at the minimum there should be 5-7 wet diapers and 3-4 soiled diapers. Some milk fed babies poop after every feeding, and some will go days without a stool. Paying attention to your child's cues will help you determine if they are constipated are experiencing discomfort.

NORMAL BOWEL MOVEMENTS

The first few poops your child has will be a green-ish black tar consistency .

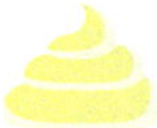

Babies who receive human milk will have yellow-ish (sometimes with hints of green or brown) poop. It can be loose, and./or seedy in appearance.

Formula feed babies will have slightly more formed poops in darker shades.

CONTACT YOUR PEDIATRICIAN

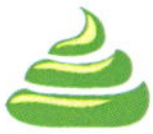

If your child's poop looks like mushy peas, it may be diarrhea and a sign they are dehydrated.

If your child's poop is white-grey or a pale black they may be experiencing issues with their liver.

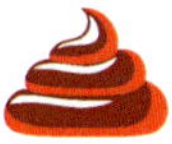

If your child's poop is reddish-brown there may be blood in their stool or they may be battling an infection.

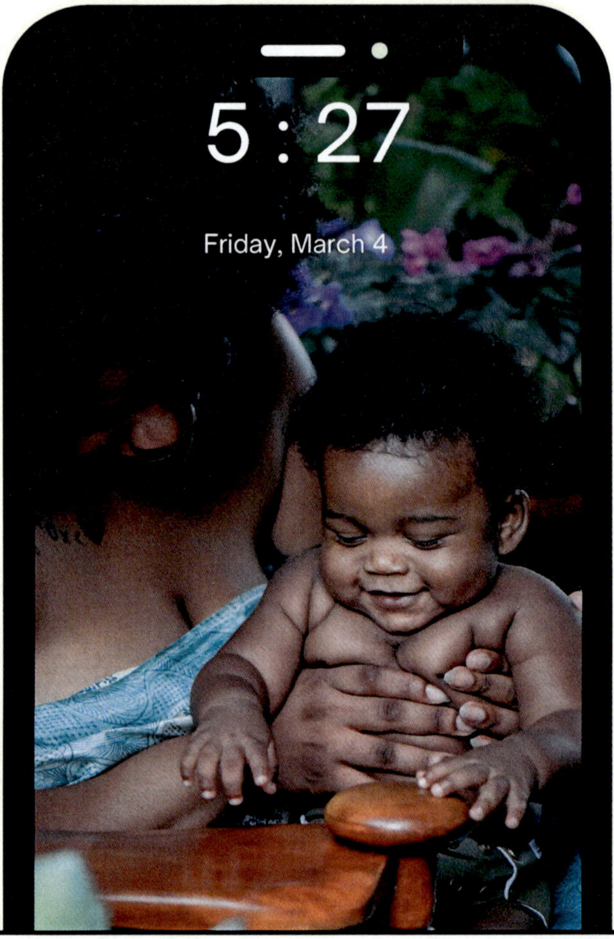

REMINDER 2m ago

Always store expressed milk in the area that gets the least amount of air exposure.

- **WITHIN 3-6 HOURS ROOM**
- **WITHIN 2-5 DAYS REFRIGERATOR**
- **WITHIN 6-9 MONTHS FREEZER**

FREEZING MILK

Pumped milk will vary in color and consistency depending on your diet and the needs of your baby. Stored milk will separate with fat rising to the top. Cool milk before freezing and store in small amounts to allow for expansion while freezing and to avoid waste. If using milk storage bags carefully lay them flat when sealing to save on storage space. When storing, label your milk with the date, if your child was sick, or if you wanted to use the milk for alternative reasons. If ice crystals are present milk can be refrozen.

THAWING MILK

There are three ways to thaw milk, first it can be placed in the refrigerator overnight. Alternatively it can be held under warm running water or placed in a container to thaw at room temperature with or without warm water. Thawed milk can be refrigerated for consumption for up to 24 hours and should NOT be refrozen. Microwaving changes the chemical composition of milk. Milk should NEVER be heated on the stove or in a microwave because it can create hot spots that can cause severe burns.

WHEN AWAY, RETURNING TO WORK

Being upfront with support staff will allow them to create the appropriate conditions for you to be comfortable.

Your pumping schedule is reflective of your child's feeding pattern. Informing your peers or colleagues may help them better understand your need to maintain a routine.

Familiarize yourself with your pump and have a packed pumping bag. It is important you develop a routine to decrease creating a stressful pumping environment.

Look at photos and videos of your child. Having a blanket, they've been wrapped in can also boost oxytocin levels and help stimulate milk production.

It's important when pumping that you are patient and kind with your body. There is so much joy in the discipline of lactation.

In all 50 states within the United States new parents have the right to a safe, private and clean pumping environment at work. When planning your maternity leave, inform HR of your plans to pump at work and ask them what arrangements they have in place.

Educators may not be able to dedicate time away from their desk. Investing in black out curtains and a small fridge can make your pumping routine more comfortable and convenient.

It's important when pumping that you are patient and kind with your body. There is so much joy in the discipline of lactation.

CAREGIVER CONDITIONS

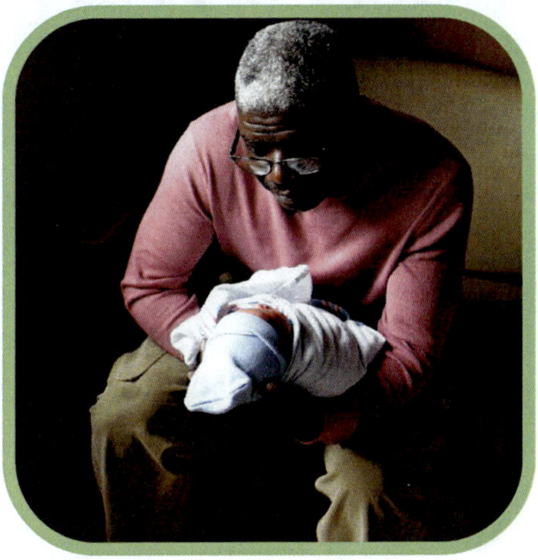

When introducing the bottle, the practice of paced feeding resembles the suckling pattern. Make sure the baby is on inclined to gravity to assist with their swallow. Practicing paced feeding prevents digestive issues and discomfort from overeating.

Talk to potential caregivers about your child's feeding schedule. This allows the caregiver to be proactive and reduce the chance of your child is distressed.

Let them know the importance of your child getting your milk. Make it clear that your child should NOT receive any formula or substitution without your permission.

WHEN TO CALL THE MIDWIFE/OB

- FEVER OF 100.4 F OR HIGHER
- PASSING LARGE CLOTS AND/OR SOAKING AN ENTIRE SANITARY NAPKIN WITHIN AN HOUR
- SWELLING, TENDERNESS OR PAIN IN YOUR LEGS
- FOUL SMELLING DISCHARGE
- CHEST PAINS, NAUSEA OR VOMITTING
- PAINFUL URINATION
- EXPERIENCING SEVERE DEPRESSION OR AUDITORY HALLUCINATIONS
- C-SECTION SCAR BECOMES RED, SWOLLEN OR DRAINS

WHEN TO CALL THE PEDIATRICIAN

- FEVER OF 100.4 F OR HIGHER
- NOT ENOUGH WET OR SOILED DIAPERS
- RED/ORANGE OR WHITISH MUCUS IN DIAPERS
- TROUBLE BREATHING
- BLUISH OR YELLOWISH SKIN TINT
- POOR APPETITE
- PROJECTILE VOMITTING
- REDNESS/SWELLING OR PUS FROM UMBILICAL CORD

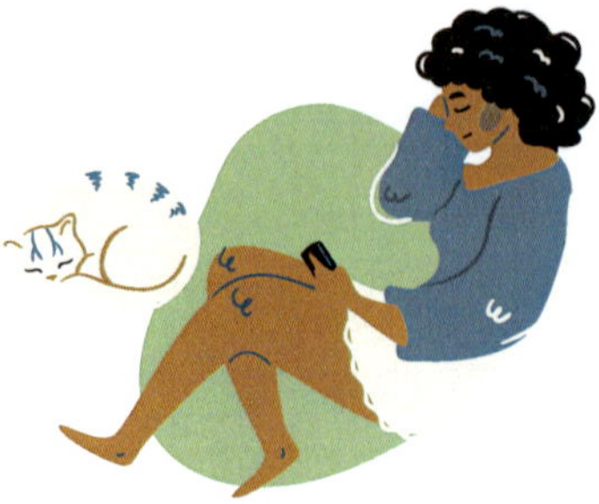

REST

Honor your journey. Acknowledging what your body has accomplished means giving your vessel grace to rest in admiration.

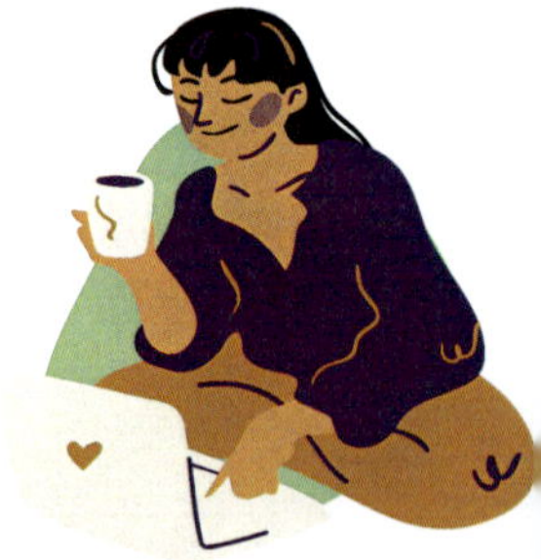

RELAX

Time desires to support you. Be present to the experiences of your journey because they are opportunities to love yourself and others deeply.

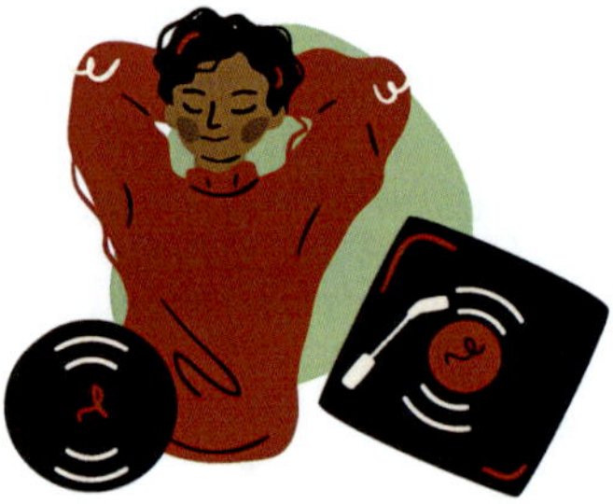

RISE

Discover new ways to celebrate your authenticity, you are more than enough, even if you may feel different.

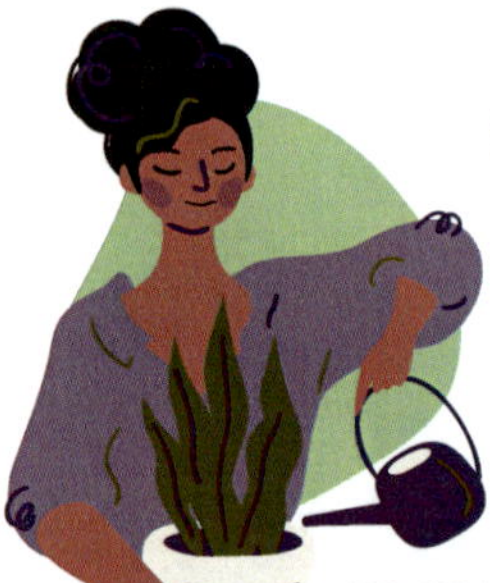

ROUTINE

Find joy in the discipline of showing up for yourself. It can be as simple as a daily word of kindness, but consistency is important.

EVERY DROP
NOURISHES.

TIME
SUPPORTS YOU,

AND,
YOU ARE ENOUGH.

Made in United States
North Haven, CT
15 July 2024

54817929R00024